Metamorphosis

Also by Judith McDaniel

November Woman
Winter Passage
The Stories We Hold Secret: Tales of Women's Spiritual Development
  (coeditor)
Sanctuary, A Journey

Metamorphosis
Reflections on Recovery

by
Judith McDaniel

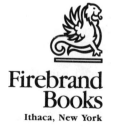

Firebrand
Books
Ithaca, New York

This book may not be reproduced, in whole or in part, except in the case
of reviews, without permission from Firebrand Books, 141 The Commons,
Ithaca, New York 14850.

Book and cover design by Mary A. Scott
Cover art by Ashley Miller
Typesetting by Bets Ltd.

Printed in the United States on acid-free paper by McNaughton & Gunn.

Library of Congress Card No. 89–080611

for the women traveling the same road

Contents

Struggle and Recovery

Struggle and Recovery:
A Feminist Looks At Twelve-Step Programs

*The awful daring of a moment's surrender
which an age of prudence can never retract.*
T.S. Eliot

Anonymity is one of the cornerstones of the Twelve-Step programs. According to this tradition as it is generally understood, if I were going to write about my own recovery, I would have to publish this work as Judith M. If I were to discuss Twelve-Step programs in the abstract as a professional, I could list my full name and speak in the third person about "a woman's recovery." One of the things I like about the Twelve-Step programs and the development of the Twelve-Step traditions, however, is that there is space for individual discernment.

I do intend both to write about my own recovery from alcoholism and to analyze how women fare in Twelve-Step programs. But I do not write as a professional in the field of alcoholism, and I do not pretend to represent A.A. or any other Twelve-Step program. I am a poet, not an alcoholism counselor. And I am an alcoholic who struggles with recovery, not a "cured" alcoholic who is going to tell you how wonderful or perfect my recovery has been. What I have written is personal, eclectic, and totally unsupported by statistics, surveys, or other social scientific apparatus. I hope, instead, to bring you the truth of poetry and the witness of an individual life in struggle.

As I approach this discussion, I feel I need to make several other assumptions overt and specific. The only Twelve-Step program I know well is Alcoholics Anonymous. I have been to an occasional Al-Anon meeting (originally, the program developed for those who lived closely with an alcoholic), but I have not attended any of the other Twelve-Step programs which are not based on the presumption of a physical addiction. It is important to me to make this distinction between physical addiction and addictions based in behavior. I understand that there are similarities, but for me to say that I am powerless over alcohol is to describe a physical addiction which results in certain psychological and behavioral adaptations. I believe that is different from the process of repeating behavioral patterns until they become second nature and can then be called addictions.

I also come to this discussion as a feminist. I assume that feminism is a context out of which I process information from my environment. Twelve-Step programs are similar in this respect. Neither contains a set of conclusions; each stresses examining and understanding experience. Feminism, however, also connects the examination of personal experience to the structures which define our lives—structures like patriarchy and capitalism—and out of these connections we derive some of the political generalities that are popularly referred to as feminism.

> *Thoughts that do often lie too deep for tears. . . .*
> W. Wordsworth

Journal Entry, 3 July 1977

I said on July 1st that I wasn't going to drink for thirty days. Janice had said that if I tried it I would learn some interesting things. That night she and Peter were coming to dinner and the first thing I learned was that I was embarrassed for her to know I was trying it. So I had a beer and some wine and since I was going to Wisconsin the next day I told myself I didn't want to do it on my last evening with Maureen and be nervous and irritable and besides Dad's call had upset me—that Mother was worse and they were both despondent. So last night I was going to start, but Dad had a bottle of his Arkansas wine open and so I had two glasses of that. And what I am learning, I think, is that I can always find a good reason not to stop. And that social pressure

to drink is everywhere, even here at home where
they do it so seldom. Perhaps today will be day one.

In fact, it took more than four years for day one to become
day two, for day two to become a month, then two, then more.
Not easily, and not in an unbroken sequence. When, in De-
cember of 1983, I began writing the poems that constitute
Metamorphosis I had been sober for nearly one year.

The first poem that came to me was "The Doe," a poem about
being alone in my life and experiencing all of that interior space
as emptiness, as loss so painful it was as if parts of my body
had been amputated—like the deer's foreleg was shot off. Out
of that apparent void, however, I was able to begin to work
on a long poem which described those last years of drinking.
I was trying to understand—insofar as understanding is
possible—why it happened and what it meant. "The Descent"
is that poem.

> She drank when she was tired for the strength
> to see her through, she drank when she was angry
> for the strength to hold it back, she drank
> when she felt strongly so the feeling wouldn't
> show, she drank when she felt nothing
> to bring the feeling back. She
> drank when she was the only one, the different
> one, the one who had to make the difference
> who had to lead the way, who showed where
> to begin. She drank when being different
> made others feel afraid, left her standing
> all alone. . . .
>   And when she had to shut
> them out she drank and when she had to go
> out to meet them she drank and when
> she drank she thought it was they who
> would not let her in.
>   So that the rooms
> grew darker and the air she breathed seemed
> to have all been breathed before.

"The Descent" also recorded the physical addiction and the experience of attempting to overcome it.

> I shook all day of the night
> I went to talk about how maybe
> I was ready to think about
> not drinking. I'd been alone
> for two weeks, told myself I didn't
> have a problem. Others made it up.
> And if no one was there to see
> I'd find my natural level. I did.
> And couldn't breathe at all when
> I woke up. I was scared.
> Scared. I didn't know why
> but I was shaking inside and it
> worked its way out to my hands
> and my voice when I spoke. All day
> I said, hey, it's nothing to be
> afraid of, and I was afraid.
> I'd thought that death was the end
> of changing, but this change
> felt like death. . . .

> We each come differently to that place
> where there is nothing left. We reach out
> to touch firm ground and find
> we've already gone down further even
> than that and there is no room to turn,
> to shift, no room to move at all
> or breathe. The earth sat on her chest
> like yesterday's promises.

We each come differently to that place where there is nothing left.
What does it mean to have an addiction? To me it meant being so focused on my substance, alcohol, that there was no space left for anything else. All of the interests, passions, pursuits of my life which defined me, let me know myself as an adult person, were pushed out of my life. And it meant doing

things that my adult self did not recognize as me, actions that were contradictory to those values I had thought were mine, those values I assumed were part of who I was, actions that were even contrary to common sense and intelligence.

Recognizing the addiction and the behavior which accompanies a physical addiction is what the First Step is about: *We admitted we were powerless over alcohol—that our lives had become unmanageable.*[1] In psychology, an overwhelming feeling of powerlessness is sometimes referred to as the ego death which precedes a rapid and apparently spontaneous transformation of the personality. Ego death is a condition of profound alienation, a circumstance well-known to alcoholics who have hit bottom.

Liberation theologian Dorothee Soelle calls this condition of alienation a death of the spirit, or "death by bread alone." To live by bread alone, she says, "is to die a slow and dreadful death in which all human relationships are mutilated and strangled." In this state the body still seems to function, and we go, more or less, about our daily business.

Soelle uses an image from a Beckett play, *Happy Days*, to describe this death by bread alone. "There is a character by the name of Winnie, a woman of about fifty," in the play. "In the first act Winnie is buried in sand up to her waist; nonetheless she chatters away, brushes her teeth, rummages about in her handbag, and feels sorry for her husband. In the second act she is buried up to her chin and can no longer move her head. All relationships are severed, but that stream of idle chatter, in which she takes herself so seriously, flows on and on . . . ."

Soelle continues her description, and those who are familiar with the disease of alcoholism—or other physical addictions—will find something familiar in this litany. "Death by bread alone means being alone and then wanting to be left alone; being friendless, yet distrusting and despising others and then being forgotten; living only for ourselves and then feeling unneeded; being unconcerned about others and wanting no one to be concerned about us; neither laughing or being laughed at; neither crying for another nor being cried for by another."[2]

We each come differently to that
place where there is nothing left. We reach out
to touch firm ground and find
we've already gone down further even
than that and there is no room to turn,
to shift, no room to move at all
or breathe. The earth sat on her chest
like yesterday's promises.

There is a hidden danger in alcoholism, I think, and perhaps in other addictions also. It has to do with "yesterday's promises." The alienation that Dorothee Soelle is describing is the result of the structures of violence in our society which separate us from one another. If we live in that condition of alienation, we will love or desire or pursue obsessively anything which gives us a feeling of connection to ourselves, to one another, to our environment. And when it is no longer possible to get that high of warmth and connection from alcohol, we will still drink because it at least takes away the pain of our loss, numbs us to our condition of alienation.

For a while, alcohol was a gift for many of us. It was for me. I will never be able to forget my first drink. A lonely, isolated teenager who did not understand that my lesbian sexuality made me a misfit in teenage dating/mating rituals, I usually hung out on the edge of a crowd, nervous, awkward. One night, ostensibly no different from any other, I went along with a group after a movie. We were all children of military personnel stationed abroad, and so we went off base to a wine cellar in Wiesbaden, Germany. When the other kids ordered beer and wine, I did too. I liked the sweet flowery taste of the wine, and I liked how I began to feel. I felt like I belonged, like I was part of a crowd, a community, if you will. For those moments, the wine solved my alienation; it eased my pain; it showed me—like a promise—*how* being part of a community could feel. From listening to other women's stories, I now know that you didn't have to be lesbian in order not to fit into an insane and misogynist socialization process. We all—those of us who became addicted—used alcohol to ease the pain, to *be* the person we longed to be, the person we had a right to be. But alcohol doesn't solve things. It only puts the promises off indefinitely.

> and yet for her the old ways led
> only to that place where there was nothing
> left and when she came to that place
> she knew it now for what it was
> and turning she began the journey out.

Knowing an addiction for what it is, that is the First Step. And we take it many times. Those of us who have experienced addiction know that we found ourselves over and over in that place "where there was nothing left." If it had been possible to change because we wanted to change, we would have done so. Some of us changed everything else—lovers, jobs, homes, friends—hoping to shake the physical addiction. Some of us experienced the loss of everything we valued, believed we wanted out of life. And we knew we were losing those things because of our drinking, our addiction, but could see no way to make it different. We were, we believed, victims of life, victims of other people, especially of those people we had trusted to take care of us.

How did it change? The turning nearly defies description, the turning away from the old ways of addiction, the turning to begin the journey out. The Second Step tells us we *came to believe a Power greater than ourselves could restore us to sanity.*

Poet Joan Larkin describes the turning as "a vision," as if

> a bell hung in my heart
> a bell of feeling
> glowed in me
> then the silence   peace
> it was then I got sober
> after a vision you have to do it
> so the next one can come to you.[3]

It is possible, I believe, that only poetry can describe and amplify the Second Step, since it is not really a step, but a leap. For me, it was a huge leap of faith that changed every aspect of the landscape of my life. I cannot explain how it happened. Probably it was the accumulation of effort after effort, a gradual movement toward an edge I couldn't even see. And then one day I had gone over it. The poem "The Earthquake" expressed the feeling of Step Two for me.

I sat up waking
and felt newness
in the still darkened
air   then the earth
trembled   not tentative
but a deepdown rumble
was shaking every surface
and I felt the rocks
shifting and my house
rattling as the earth's
bones readjusted.

When it was quiet
I thought   now they will see
the surface all the same
but underneath I know
every rock and fissure
each line of stress and weakness
has been rearranged and lives
in new relationship   each to each.

When I experienced the actual earthquake in the poem, I was still living with my lover in the home we had built together. I had been sober for four or five months and was very aware that my life was different, even if I couldn't say exactly what else had changed. At the surface level, the only thing that had changed between my lover and me was the ritual of a before-dinner drink, wine with dinner. And yet, I knew it was different. Something deep within me, unnameable at first, had been touched, like the bedrock beneath the earth had been touched. But only I knew. Writing the poem was a recognition of that knowing.

It is important to notice that there are two intertwining strands occurring simultaneously in Step Two. Not only do we need to stop drinking, we need to be *restored to sanity*. We have to desire sanity as well as the life-saving relief of not drinking alcoholically. Many of us know former drunks who have given up alcohol and changed nothing else in their lives, who have been unable to alter the patterns of insanity that compulsive drinking induces. Step Two is simple and mysterious. It requires an action—desiring sanity—and then a surrender—letting the change, the bedrock shift, happen.

And that is the process of recovery described in Steps One and Two. First is the recognition and then the willingness to accept change, to accept where the understanding has led us. Those two Steps happen both to women and to men, I think, with the same frequency, but never with the same impact from one woman to the next or one man to the next; each experience of the turning is totally unique to the individual and completely similar in its transformative power.

The difficulty for me—and for many women with whom I talk or to whom I listen in A.A. Meetings year after year, however—is what comes next, Step Three: we *made a decision to turn our will and our lives over to the care of God as we understood* Him.

One of my difficulties with all of the Steps, and this Step stands out for me, is the language. Language is important to me. I am a poet and I have nearly stopped apologizing for caring about the language. So I have to try to ignore the use of male pronouns . . . both for the alcoholic and for god. I have to substitute the actual word *god* for *him* when I read the literature. Some women use *god as we understand her*. But I believe in an enspirited universe, and my god concept refuses to be identified by anthropomorphic pronouns of either gender. Some of us doggedly refer to our "higher power" and others use the collective power of the group as our higher power. One friend insists that her higher power is her Marxist philosophy, and another just as adamantly maintains her higher power is Beethoven, since listening to his music empowers her. Like many women, I have stretched to make this program work for me because I have needed it. And today it sometimes seems to me that the founders of A.A. may not have known *why* their program worked.

For example, in the book *Alcoholics Anonymous* which explains the history of A.A. and how the program works, Bill W. talks about the necessity of Step Three—*made a decision to turn our will and our lives over to the care of God*—because of "self-will run riot." Alcoholics, he says, have thought only of themselves, of what would please or suit themselves during their drinking years, and Step Three is salutary, reminding alcoholics, "not my will, but thine." Well, in my years in A.A. I have seen women alcoholics who fit that description as it is written. But far more often I have seen women who have been trapped in lives against their wills, women who have had no say in the conditions of their lives, who have never had a chance to exercise self-will at all, let alone experience "self-will run riot." Conventional A.A. wisdom tells us that this step is necessary to make alcoholics "educable," willing to change; humility, we are told, is the state of mind in which education for change can begin to work.

How, I asked myself in those first months and years when I was struggling to stay sober, am I to accept the conventional (read white-heterosexual-Christian-male) interpretation for myself and other women? I did, on occasion, get downright nasty over this. In my second year of recovery I went to a retreat on Women and Alcohol sponsored by a local Dominican Retreat Center. I was O.K. with the fact that the retreat was being led by a priest, I told myself, because most of the time we would be in discussion groups and they would be made up of women. But I was not a happy camper when the retreat opened on Friday night and the only recovering alcoholics invited to speak were men—the priest and a friend of his. And I was even less thrilled the next day when the discussion of Step Three focused around this issue of educability, and we were all told to go off in our discussion groups and consider humility and how we could achieve it. I had been listening to these women talk all evening and morning about the conditions of their lives. Some had lost children because of our disease; most of us had lost significant relationships, or careers, or our jobs, our chance for independence. We shared the humiliation of hitting bottom —and for many of us only part of that hitting bottom was the result of our alcoholism.

While I do understand that men hit bottom too, and that it can be a profoundly humiliating experience, I need to suggest that *how* white middle- and upper-class heterosexual men *experience* that hitting bottom is different from how women or gay people or people of color experience it. Because for the most part they have experienced their right to choose for themselves, to exercise self-will very differently from nondominant members of this society. And so that day, before we broke into discussion groups, I suggested to the priest that perhaps his experience was not the only one we should be listening to, perhaps the women there in that room knew for ourselves what we needed in order to be receptive to education for change. For myself, I said, I needed to talk about self-esteem, not humility. I needed to believe that my life, that *I*, was important enough, mattered enough to struggle for. As women, I said, we have all spent a great deal of time struggling for others' survival needs. One of the first lessons feminism taught us was that we need to struggle for ourselves in order to have anything authentic to offer others. So I led a discussion group on self-esteem. But I left the retreat early and went home, carrying with me the nagging feeling that I was missing some basic connection.

Years later, I think I understand that connection. Humility is not the acceptance of humiliation, allowing others to humiliate us or indulging in self-humiliation. Humility has its source in the word *humus*, of the earth, grounded. Humility, then, is an accurate and honest assessment of who we are; this assessment will include knowing our strengths and our weaknesses. For women, this usually means acknowledging and acting on our strengths, since many of us have felt ourselves to be victims of our lives and have experienced our weaknesses over and over. And so I was right. Women do need to talk about self-esteem. We need to understand the power we *do* have, and to discuss in safe places ways in which we can exercise that power in the world. It is an essential precondition to going out in the world and being self-empowered.

In one publication written on this difficult Third Step, the author suggests that "short of a miracle blessing us with a sudden conversion experience, carrying out the decision to turn our wills and lives over is a daily, life-long process. If we could accomplish a complete turnover at this point, the Twelve Steps could be reduced to Three Steps and ongoing involvement in the program would not be necessary."[4] If that is true, if the remaining nine Steps are intended to facilitate the process of "turning it over," perhaps we can better understand the function of Step Three by looking at the Steps that follow.

> *. . .even*
> *my tools are the wrong ones*
> *for what I have to do.*
> Adrienne Rich

Steps Four through Ten are aimed, I believe, at making us fit to live with—to live with ourselves and to live in the world. That was not, however, my first response to these Steps and their language, a language that is—throughout all Twelve Steps—fiercely theological, restrictively patriarchal and Christian. My own coming to terms with Steps Four through Ten was difficult. I knew the Steps were working in my life, helping me to live with more sanity and purpose, making my work more focused and my relationships more caring. Yet, they embarrassed me, the Twelve Steps. I wanted to apologize for them to my friends who were not in A.A. I wanted to fix them when we read them in women's meetings. Ultimately, this search for a better word or a better way led me, not to apology, but to reconciliation. The language was not written the way I would have written it, but the process was taking me in a direction I desperately wanted to go.

For example, Step Four asks us to make *a searching and fearless moral inventory* of ourselves and then, in Step Five, we admit *to God, to ourselves, and to another human being the exact nature of our wrongs.* When I first read those Steps I knew I could never be a part of this program. Not only was I not a Christian, I wasn't a Catholic; and I knew a confession when I saw one. But I hadn't counted on how hard it is to get rid of a physical addiction, that continual gnawing awareness that every cell in my body wanted a drink. I had to talk about *that* with other women who knew what I was experiencing. So I kept going to meetings. Gradually the actuality of Steps Four and Five transcended the language in which they were written.

As I sat week after week in a circle of women at my A.A. meeting listening to the stories of their lives, telling my own stories, I was reminded of the feminist process of Consciousness Raising groups. Those of us who have been a part of a C.R. group understand how necessary it is to speak our own realities out loud. Talking about our lives, seeing that others accept our truths as we say them, is incredibly self-empowering. What we learned in those groups was that sharing our secrets was one way to disallow their power over us. Usually in the telling of what we have hidden we discover that others have had experiences similar to our own, that we are not alone. My secret—that I craved alcohol beyond reason or explanation—was not shameful in an A.A. context. That discovery is part of the healing, part of the recovery.

I will admit that I have not taken Step Five literally. I have done an inventory of my strengths and weaknesses, but the only god to whom I have admitted them is "that of god in everyone."[5] It has been enough for me to tell my secrets to women like me, women who understand because they have lived the same secrets, experienced the same terror when we could no longer control our drinking or the things we did when we were drinking.

The function of Steps Six and Seven is profound change, and once again it took me years to understand—in that place deep within and beyond language—what they were really about. In Step Six we become willing to change (*were entirely ready to have God remove all these defects of character*) and in Seven ask that our shortcomings, the ones we have named for ourselves, be removed (*humbly asked him to remove our shortcomings*).

One of the several recent criticisms of A.A. published in the lesbian and gay press cites Step Seven, in particular, as an example of how A.A. "insures the timidity and passivity" of lesbians who are involved in its program.[6] I understand that it can be hard to see how Steps Six and Seven are anything but an encouragement to passivity. Why don't we just rewrite them, as another critic suggests, and say that "we discovered we could use this power inside us to overcome our alcoholism . . . ."[7]

The assumption being made by both of these writers, it seems to me, is that if we want to change, we can just change. We are strong women. We have the power to do that, don't we?

The truth is that change is often not this simple. Why would we cling to a behavior that we abhorred, that harmed us and those we loved? Perhaps because it is known, familiar.

Writing about a different kind of recovery in my poem "Leaving Home," I discovered that sometimes

> . . .Grief can be a cushion.
> You sink down and down into the familiarity of it and when it starts to feel normal, comfortable even, then it's time to look for a horizon of bare rock and blasted trees, anything less familiar where you can hear all the words sharp and clear.[8]

Pain, too, can be a cushion; destructive behavior as well. We are drawn to the familiarity of what we have known, and anything new and unknown can seem more frightening than the hell we may presently be living in. Being willing to change takes tremendous courage and energy. Naming the changes we want to make, taking responsibility for how we want to be in the world, carries the willingness into action. The character defects we are asking to be removed are the same ones we identified for ourselves in Step Four. No one waves a magic wand over some vague, unspecified thing that is wrong with us. We do it: we become willing and then we step toward an uncharted future.

Steps Eight and Nine move those interior changes out into the world: we *made a list of all persons we had harmed,* particularly during our active alcoholism, and then we *made direct amends to such people wherever possible.* As we begin to consider the people we may have harmed, it is natural that we look also at the things that harmed *us,* those conditions of alienation every alcoholic has known. Part of making amends always requires that we make amends to ourselves, recognize the ways in which we were hurt, the damage we sustained, the structures and systems that harmed us.

I believe Steps Eight and Nine ensure that alcoholics can no longer consider themselves victims. In these Steps we say, yes, we have been harmed by alcohol; but we ultimately are required to take responsibility for our actions, the positive and the negative, the sober and the drunk.

When I was very new in sobriety I began to experience the disintegration of the long-term primary relationship in my life. Of course, I experienced that disintegration as *happening* to me. I felt I was the victim of my lover's decision to leave. Her leaving seemed a violation of my very core being, an ultimate betrayal of our years of loving and trusting.

The pain that went along with being a victim was familiar to me, and I was no stranger to self-righteousness of the "how could she do this to me?" variety. But there was something wrong with this picture. For nearly a year, during the last months of my drinking, I had been contributing to the disintegration of our relationship. I didn't mean to. I didn't want to. I would have given just about anything not to have done it. At some level, though, I wasn't in control. And so for nearly a year I had had an affair, and I lied when my lover asked me about it, denied to her over and over that it was happening.

At some point, before she left and after our relationship was over, I knew I had to tell her what had happened during that year. I thought I was doing it for her, giving her back her own sense of reality. I felt scared, but also generous and self-sacrificing, as we sat down to talk. When the conversation was over, however, I was devastated when I discovered the result: I could not tell a single friend what was happening to me without admitting my own participation in the breakup. "Poor me" became an impossibility. I was allowed my pain; it was real and it hurt.

But the slogan I heard over and over in A.A. meetings at this time was "Pain is inevitable, suffering is optional." Pain, they were telling me, is a feeling, and anger is a feeling. But self-pity and blaming others for my situation were attitudes, and I could change them with a little work. My A.A. friends were trying to let me know I wasn't a victim, that I was an actor in the process. I was responsible, and ultimately that responsibility has been empowering.

Step Ten is a transition Step which brings us into the present. Step Ten demands that we keep on learning and practicing the process of honest assessment and redirection by continuing *to take personal inventory and when we were wrong promptly admitted it*. This is a maintenance Step, one that acknowledges we will continue to make mistakes, experience conflict, want more than we can achieve.

Steps Ten, Eleven, and Twelve make of this process a spiral rather than a closed circle. Without them the concept of a Twelve-Step program would be stultifying and would probably have never become more than a cult for a few. Step Ten insists that we live in the present, not in the mistakes of the past. Step Eleven says we must continue to improve our spiritual life (*improve our conscious contact with God as we understood Him*). And Step Twelve requires us to take the learning out into the world, *to carry this message to alcoholics, and to practice these principles in all our affairs*.

As I worked through these Steps and the process of reconciliation I described earlier, I began to realize there are several assumptions about our relationship to our own experience
and the structures that created it which are embedded in the
Twelve Steps, assumptions that are important to me as a woman and feminist trying to use A.A. One assumption is that
honesty in our own self-analysis—no matter how painful—will
aid our transformation from addiction to sobriety *and* that honesty in dealing with our environment will enhance our lives
in the long term.

Most important, as I have been discussing, are some of the
assumptions about power and control contained in the Steps.
Powerlessness is not good. That is what we are when we are
drinking or drugging. Recognizing and admitting powerlessness
is, however, essential to changing our condition. We are asked
to take control of our own actions—taking an inventory, making amends, sharing the message—but we are asked, at the
same time, to turn our life and our will over to that god of our
understanding. The A.A. slogan which attempts to explain this
apparent contradiction is "You can plan actions, you can't plan
outcomes." In other words, I can take responsibility by making amends to someone; I cannot ensure how my amends will
be taken, cannot ensure there will be a specific outcome that
will please me. I have no power to make someone else be the
way I want her to be.

Discussions of power and powerlessness, of self-empowerment versus power over others, have been central to feminism.
I don't think that the assumptions about power contained in
the Twelve Steps are antithetical to those of feminism. Sug-
gestions, therefore, that Twelve-Step programs (and not Ronald
Reagan) have destroyed radical feminism, or that the lesbian
community has fallen prey to a fundamentalist cult, seem mis-
guided to me. I don't believe, in the final analysis, that a responsible reading of the Twelve Steps will lead to the conclusion
that they advocate powerlessness.

I do remember, however, my own first response to the language of A.A. and I know I was not positively impressed by

a Step that asked me, as Step Three did, *to turn our will and our lives over to the care of God as we understood Him.* Isn't this an acceptance of powerlessness? A rationalization for passivity? I wondered. If I turn myself over to this higher power, haven't I then been absolved of responsibility? It's not me who has to make the world a fit place to live in. Let the higher power take care of it.

But there are several other ways to consider the issues raised by Step Three. The first is that the equation of power with control is a socialized one. We assume that power means control because we have been taught so within a contemporary Western patriarchal school of thought. There are other philosophical approaches that teach very different ideas about power and self-empowerment, schools of thought in which giving up the idea that we are in control of every element of our lives does not mean giving up our own power to initiate or respond. In addition, I do not myself believe we have all power within us; and on some occasions I see nothing wrong or weak in calling upon an energy that is beyond me.

The Twelve Steps assume that human beings are spiritual beings. We may each have a very different understanding of what this means, but the Twelve-Step program is premised on the belief that if we don't nurture that part of us, we will not achieve our goal of sobriety, of living whole. To me, living whole means acknowledging my deep connection to all life and, at the same time, being astonished by my own uniqueness, by something that

> . . .was with me from the first
> some impulse, some stance, some way of beginning
> that roots this life against the precipice,
> that curls—a tight fisted seed—waiting,
> always waiting for the fire's clean sweep.[9]

The polarization of human and animal, body and soul, intellect and spirit, politics and spirituality—this polarization is, once again, Western and patriarchal. I will not choose between political involvement and spiritual enhancement, between a life which challenges my mind or one which nourishes my heart/emotions/soul. These are false choices, choices we make when we accept the definitions created by the society that has also created our profound alienation from one another and our own sources of being. Poet Audre Lorde has reminded us, in another context, that "the master's tools will never dismantle the master's house."[10] If we, as feminists, insist on using only patriarchal definitions of power and self-empowerment in our discussions, our formulations, we will never be able to build new and liberating concepts.

Having said that, however, I also believe it is important to acknowledge that any transformative learning process can be corrupted into a disempowering process, particularly if the goal of transformative change becomes instead a prescription for a specific, already identified outcome. I have, for example, experienced varieties of feminism that described "successful liberation" as corporate or academic success. Those models seem as stifling to me as the pre-liberation ideas of what a woman "should be." And I do know A.A. meetings in which the interpretation of the Twelve Steps seems to me stifling and proscriptive, in which dependency on the group or individuals in the group does create a closing off of vision rather than an opening into the world. I have known women who traded their dependency on drugs and alcohol for dependency on an A.A. group. Ultimately, however, I believe this is a less destructive dependency because it leaves the woman alive for potential future growth and change.

But I am surely not advocating reading Step Three as an encouragement to passivity. It simply wouldn't be consistent with what we find in all of the other Steps. In them we are asked to be an active participant in our own lives. We are asked, on a daily basis, to look at ourselves, our relationships, the circumstances under which we live and work, and we are asked to be honest, to be open to change, to be caring for those who suffer as we have. Can we not try to read Step Three in a way that is in keeping with these values embedded in the other Steps?

For me, the essential realization was that if I were going to live in my world as an involved and self-empowered person, I was committing myself to inevitable struggle. I wrote about this in an essay on the Women's Peace Encampment at Seneca Falls. The experience of the encampment was not a peaceful one, not for women who participated, not for the townspeople of the local villages. But I understood that something very important had taken place in that atmosphere of stress and challenge: education for transformation. In my own experience, I remembered that "my most important learning has taken place *not* when I was most comfortable, not even when I was sort of comfortable, but when I was dragged kicking and screaming through some of the most painful experiences of my life."[11]

Turning it over—as we are asked to do in Step Three, I would suggest—is not a calm and graceful process, although it may eventually be grace-filled. Turning it over does not mean an end to struggle. For example, it does not mean I will never experience again the desire to drink. Four years sober, I found myself sitting at a business lunch with colleagues. I was facing the bar and I watched across the room as the bartender put two brandy snifters up on the counter, reached—almost in slow-motion, it seemed now—for the brandy bottle, and poured the golden amber brandy into the glasses. My heart was beating slowly and very deeply as I saw this. I couldn't drag my eyes away from those glasses, and as I watched the brandy started to shimmer and glow and pulse with life, as vivid a hallucination as I'd ever had when I was drinking. Did I want a drink in that moment? Oh, yes, like few other things I have ever wanted. Did I have to struggle, painfully, to excuse myself from lunch and leave that place? Yes, of course.

Taking Step Three means to me that I have committed myself to that struggle. Turning it over does not mean it will be easy, or that I can be a passive observer to my own life. Turning it over means letting myself be led to be the best person

30

I can be, not the most politically correct, not the most nice, but letting myself be drawn repeatedly into the life-affirming process of struggling to become myself.

Turning it over means acknowledging the incredible alienation fostered by the social systems in which we live and working to create community in spite of it. Turning it over means affirming "yesterday's promises," those promises we sensed early on in our experiences with alcohol, promises of connection to one another, deep connectedness to ourselves and our own experience. Because what I have learned from my years of recovery is that the struggle is what creates community, and the community in turn creates the healing that is recovery.

Unlike other afflictions in my life, alcoholism has been both a burden I have struggled with and a gift. It was at an A.A. meeting that a woman quoted Denise Levertov's poem "Stepping Westward" to me:

> If I bear burdens
>
> they begin to be remembered
> as gifts, goods, a basket
>
> of bread that hurts
> my shoulders but closes me
>
> in fragrance. I can
> eat as I go.[12]

My own alcoholism has been a gift when it allowed me, through the deep connection of my own experience, to know how someone else felt who was suffering. That gift is possible, I believe, because of the community created and supported by Twelve-Step programs. From the outside, it may not be obvious that there is community in an A.A. meeting. What, after all, do those diverse and unrelated humans have in common? Not similar interests, not geography, not faith or religious beliefs, not political commitment. What makes community here is the shared experience of an addiction that caused each of us great pain and a recovery that is possible primarily in the presence of one another as we witness our mutual change and development.

Turning it over is not an act of giving up or an act of alienation; it is, rather, a recognition that creating ourselves—and creating a world our selves would want to live in—is a life-long process. We need guidelines, those Steps that follow Step Three, so that we can live the process today, rather than waiting to live in a perfect world.

> It is difficult
> to get the news from poems
> yet men die miserably every day
> for lack
> of what is found there.
> William Carlos Williams

In order to talk about that process in *Metamorphosis*, I used the Medieval concept of *totentanz*, the deep, elusive belief that hope is somehow embedded in the most despairing of circumstances. The protagonist of this poem is, however, experiencing the despair of her own alienation, seeing only the horrible things in the world and her apparent inability to affect anything, make anything better. I called that poem "Deathdance" and it told how

> She had no heart
> for the *totentanz*
> did not understand
> how in the plague years
> the few survivors
> joined hands and danced
> among the graves and back
> to the village.
> She saw only
> the wolves
> salivating
> on the hardpacked
> snow.

But later in the sequence I was working on a poem about the process of turning it over, of committing ourselves to the struggle, and I asked a friend of mine, an older German woman who is a classics scholar, whether there was such a thing as a *lebenstanz*, a lifedance, which would express another aspect of that elusive sense of struggle and recovery we sometimes call hope. Her response became the headnote for the poem "Lebenstanz."

> Is there a lebenstanz? No no.
> That is the work we do every day.

In a blizzard she climbed
the hill   wind sucking
at her breath and the snow
icing against her eyes
as she bent her head to walk
forward on instinct
when she could not see
the ground. . . .

To act or not to act
she climbed to find the answer
and in the climbing knew
the answer was to act as though
there were no choice   for if
she believed in the circle—
that as the fossil sinks then
it will rise again to the surface

so all energy comes around
—she must act as though
each day knew the circle   knew
the answer in the wind's sharp voice.
Some days she could only half believe
some days she would know it held no truth
but on the best days she worked as though
the question mattered not at all.

Turning it over, on a good day, is something we do without having to think about it. We act as though we had no choice; that is, we engage in our lives, in creating and transforming our world, without question and without hesitation. It is, perhaps, only when something in that natural process of engagement is damaged that we must think about whether we will struggle, how we will struggle, with whom we will struggle. Only as a response to this damage is it necessary to *make a decision* to turn our lives, our wills, over to this process.

I have a fantasy that I will one day write a story that is set in this country after the revolution. And the community historian will be reminiscing about how A.A. used to have this disclaimer. Those of you familiar with Twelve-Step programs will know it: "A.A. is not allied with any sect, denomination, politics, organization or institution." And so she is telling the young ones, born after the revolution, how effective this disclaimer was—not only did it keep the FBI away from A.A. groups, but many people who engaged in the process of A.A. did not understand—consciously—that they were members of a revolutionary community. And so, she tells them, the revolution began in those thousands and thousands of A.A. groups meeting all over the United States, indeed all over the world.

I probably won't write that story, because the revolution won't happen on a particular day or month or year; and I doubt if we would be able to discern exactly when it began or when it was achieved. The revolution is about the process of struggle and recovery, recovery of self and recovery of one another, of community. It is more like climbing the mountain in a blizzard; all we know is that we have to continue.

Many women are choosing to use Twelve-Step programs today. We are choosing A.A. because we want to recover. We want to recover our right to the personal choices in our lives and to the self-determination of our own political choices. We especially want to recover those characteristics that are the opposite of alienation. It is as if we were the character in the Beckett play, buried in sand up to our chins. We need to struggle to free ourselves, slowly moving, first a shoulder, pushing a little of the sand away so we can move a bit more, then freeing an elbow, a hand, finding those pieces of ourselves that can help us as we struggle.

It is a fearsome process, this recovery, because often it puts us in new territory. We call it re-covery, but most of us were never there before, and so we don't recognize the place. It isn't familiar, and the feelings we are recovering and those pieces of ourselves we are recovering, they aren't familiar either. And sometimes that makes us afraid.

I am not concerned about fear. It is, I think, a very appropriate response at times. I am concerned that we will think the fear means we are doing the wrong thing. I am concerned that we will think the pain of struggle means we are doing the wrong thing. Quite the opposite. We all know the difference between the pain of alienation and the pain of coming alive. We know the difference between the fear which means we are being smothered and the fear of excitement, the fear and excitement of discovery. "It's gonna hurt, now," warns Toni Morrison in *Beloved*. "Anything dead coming back to life hurts."[13]

My hope is that neither the fear nor the pain will lead us into creating a Twelve-Step program that is static rather than dynamic, disempowering rather than transformative. My hope is that the choices we make for our lives will reflect our understanding of struggle and recovery and the risk-taking which is required for us to be able to dance the *lebenstanz*, the lifedance, every day of our lives.

Notes

1. The Twelve Steps from *The Twelve Steps and Twelve Traditions* (New York: Alcoholics Anonymous World Services, Inc., 1953), pp. 5-9:

"Step One: We admitted we were powerless over alcohol—that our lives had become unmanageable.

Step Two: Came to believe that a power greater than ourselves could restore us to sanity.

Step Three: Made a decision to turn our will and our lives over to the care of God *as we understood Him*.

Step Four: Made a searching and fearless moral inventory of ourselves.

Step Five: Admitted to God, to ourselves, and to another human being the exact nature of our wrongs.

Step Six: Were entirely ready to have God remove all these defects of character.

Step Seven: Humbly asked Him to remove our shortcomings.

Step Eight: Made a list of all persons we had harmed, and became willing to make amends to them all.

Step Nine: Made direct amends to such people wherever possible except when to do so would injure them or others.

Step Ten: Continued to take personal inventory and when we were wrong promptly admitted it.

Step Eleven: Sought through prayer and meditation to improve our conscious contact with God *as we understood Him*, praying only for knowledge of His will for us and the power to carry that out.

Step Twelve: Having had a spiritual awakening as the result of these steps, we tried to carry this message to alcoholics, and to practice these principles in all our affairs."

2. Dorothee Soelle, *Death By Bread Alone* (Philadelphia: Fortress Press, 1978), pp. 3-4.

3. Joan Larkin, "Broken Girl," in A *Long Sound* (Penobscot, ME: Granite Press, 1986), p. 13.

4. James G. Jensen, *Step Three, Turning It Over* (Center City, MN: Hazeldon, 1980), p. 5.

5. George Fox, "Then you will come to walk cheerfully over the world, answering that of God in everyone. . . ." in Gwyn Douglas, *Apocalypse of the Word: The Life and Message of George Fox* (Richmond, IN: Friends United Press, 1986), p. 142.

6. Joan M. Ward, "Therapism and the Taming of the Lesbian Community," *Sinister Wisdom*, No. 36, Winter 1988/89, p. 38.

7. Suzanne Ray, "Re-Writing the 12 Steps," *Lesbian Contradiction*, No. 25, Winter, 1989, p. 17.

8. Judith McDaniel, "Leaving Home," in *Sanctuary: A Journey*, (Ithaca, NY: Firebrand Books, 1987), p. 24.

9. Judith McDaniel, "Grand Canyon," unpublished poem.

10. Audre Lorde, "The Master's Tools Will Never Dismantle the Master's House," in *Sister Outsider* (Freedom, CA: The Crossing Press, 1984), p. 112.

11. Judith McDaniel, "One Summer at Seneca," in *Sanctuary: A Journey*, p. 40.

12. Denise Levertov, "Stepping Westward," in *The Sorrow Dance* (New York: New Directions, 1966).

13. Toni Morrison, *Beloved* (New York: Alfred A. Knopf, 1987), p. 35.

Based on a talk written for the Women and Spirituality Conference, Colorado Springs, Colorado, April 8-9, 1988.

Metamorphosis

Prelude

Once there was a world where change
was a part of life   where today
a ship could sail across the sea
and tomorrow when they looked out
a rock crested the waves where none
had stood before and no one was amazed
and no one denied that the rock
had been a ship yesterday
and was a rock today   for all could see
the vines sprouting in profusion
out of cracks that had been a hull

and if a woman fled across a field
to escape a god or devil and when they
looked again there stood a laurel tree
it did not need to bleed and speak
for them to know how   when she could run
no farther   her soft and sweated skin
grew hard and rough like bark and her fearful
thighs grew close and from her toes roots
sprouted deep into the hard clay-packed soil

and when young Glaucus—who loved
the sea and went each day to spread his nets
on the bountiful waters—was called
by the sea gods to become one with the water
he longed for and feared this change
and cried out until the gods came
and purged his fearful mortal nature
with magic singing   nine times repeated
sang of the sea and of river water fed
from a hundred streams until he knew
himself a different kind of creature
body and spirit   a different creature.

Nine times they sang the magic songs
nine times to welcome change
nine times to dissolve
the fiber of life as it was.

The Doe

Alone in the morning then
I became a friend of the doe
who would glide at dawn through the frozen garden
pause under my window
leap the fence   flicker of white tail.

One moon bright night
a dog's raised hackle drew me
to the window to watch a mating dance
playful shadows on the snow
a movement   and then no more
at dawn   the hoofprint memory.

Today at noon in full light
the dog's hysterical baying
I run to the window knowing
it is the last day of hunting
season and she is there
totentanz
running on three legs
one foreleg shot off at the chest
she rises   pirouettes
blood on the snow
bloodshod   I see
her other front hoof shot off.
She screams I scream my voice
rising with the dog screaming
until the state trooper comes
and she is gratefully dead
and he examines the licenses
of the two men who saunter
out of the woods permitted
to shoot doe   permitted
to gut the warm carcass
and sling it in the pickup truck.

Alone in the morning then
I look at the carmine ribbon
stretching the length of the garden
vivid as a heartbeat on snow.

Deathdance

Awake and in dreams
they came to her
the children of wars
came peering
through wire
dancing in pain
down napalmed
streets no flesh
to hide
this awful
nudity—
maimed dying dead
she saw them
in news photos
"live" on TV
dying. A boy
in Tripoli caught
by shrapnel dead
in the arms of a boy
not more than ten
called a Red Cross
worker. A girl
in New York
dead in a blaze
she could not flee
caught by a dancing
flame because her leg
was chained to a ceiling
beam by her father.

Awake and in dreams
they had come to her
down the corridors
of *might have beens*
since the morning
she heard the news—
one hundred children
rescued   airlifted
dead in a plane crash.
And she knew then
despair
knew
it was the same
to act
or not to act
it ended the same
and she did not know
what to do.

She had no heart
for the *totentanz*
did not understand
how in the plague years
the few survivors
joined hands and danced
among the graves and back
to the village.
She saw only
the wolves
salivating
on the hardpacked
snow.

The Fog

I was confused that morning when I woke up because I
looked out the window and couldn't see a thing. Just
fog. All white. And I forgot what day it was. You know
how sometimes you'll wake up and feel scared or anxious
but you don't know why. That's the worst feeling. Not
knowing. Like being a child again. For three or four
minutes I looked out at the fog and I couldn't tell
what time of year it was or even what time of day. Then
I knew. I knew everything at once. It was the first
of September and I had set the alarm early so I could jog
before she came to move her things out of the house.
I wanted to look once more at familiar things and then leave
before she came to take what she thought was hers, leave
what she thought was mine.

I was confused that morning because for nearly a year
now I had been waking up without the fog. Some
headaches at first, but no hangovers. No memory loss.
No blackouts. No fog in the brain. I could wake up knowing
what day it was and where I was and what I was going
to do and I could even remember what I had done
the day before. A celebration. When I thought about
it—waking up nearly three hundred mornings in a row
without the fog—I couldn't help smiling. So what I
wanted that day was a celebration but what I got
was a funeral. She was leaving. She said it wasn't
working for her anymore. For weeks I worried that the
other fog had come back because I listened so hard to
what she said, but still I didn't know why she was leaving.

So I put coffee on the stove, laced my jogging shoes
and let my feet find their own way up the road. Nothing
clear. Not a single outline. Just a big mushy blur.
Then out of the corner of my eye I saw something move.
Barely a warning and a huge dog looms out of the mist
looking like he's all chest and head. I know him. He
knows me. Nothing to be afraid of except how different
it all is this morning. What if I ran back down this road
and the real world moved ten years on while I was out here
in this fog? What if I ran back and found the real me
already sitting on the porch having breakfast and
nodding to the heifers in the pasture? There's the dog
again. Silent sentinel. And now I'm glad I'm not
a stranger coming down this pale and foggy road.

I sat on the porch with my coffee. The hills
were beginning to rise out of the mist now and next
to me on the porch railing was a cobweb spun so
spiderfine I almost touched it before I saw it. Would
have if it hadn't been for the dew caught in pale silver
drops along each thread. I reached out and touched
a strand, the farthest one from where the spider sat,
expecting she would scurry toward the pull on her
thread, but she sat, unsurprised. She must have known
it was only me. In such moments I had always been able
to sink down to a place where there weren't any words.
I knew that spider and she knew me. To be known
that way felt like love. Who could tell what this other
would be, this being alone without feeling the love.

Chassé en l'Air

They make us up
like children who dream smoke
into shapes as it struggles
to rise from the smoldering
pile of leaves
piling fantasy
upon fantasy.
Look at the witch.
No, it's a clown.
See the beautiful lady.

Such easy satisfaction
is the nature
of smoke
as it curls
obliging
each dreamer's whim.

But she longed
for the clarity of flame
the crackle of pure
scarlet and gold
each time she would
twist
reshape
puff herself into
another dreamer's
chimney.

The Descent

She lived in a time when stability
not change   was the key to safety
a time that said dismantling the missiles
and warheads was   destabilizing.
Balance   she heard them say   requires stasis
but she saw smoke hovering on the horizon
of every city she drove toward and held
in her memory   the hawk balanced
on a trembling wing   and she knew
the old tree grown rigid against the wind
was the tree that fell.
                              And yet for years
her worst nightmare found her in an unknown
future   alone without a landscape. Nothing
in that nightmare future was familiar—
nostalgia was connected to a known and vanished
past. She'd wake   touch the woman
sleeping familiarly close   and sleep again
sure the dream was just a fluke
surely   surely   she knew what her future
held   knew that potential landscape
as surely as she knew the arm she touched.

The rooms grew darker imperceptibly
the rooms in which she lived her life
and tried to build a present filled
with light. Looking back she could find
no single moment   no single room
or voice or face to mark the turning
when the circle became a spiral
when the way led only down.

I always wanted what I
was not supposed to want.
I don't remember the child
of four or five who told
the reporter she wanted
to be a boy named Tommy
and own a pet pig   but
last year my grandmother
gave me the clipping
out of the family bible
and there I was   wide-eyed
and smiling. Why not Tommy?
My script read different:
college   marry   mommy.
I tried to take the cues
that came my way
but that other me held back
clamped down tight
I waited.

She drank when she was tired for the strength
to see her through, she drank when she was angry
for the strength to hold it back, she drank
when she felt strongly so the feeling wouldn't
show, she drank when she felt nothing
to bring the feeling back. She
drank when she was the only one, the different
one, the one who had to make the difference
who had to lead the way, who showed where
to begin. She drank when being different
made others feel afraid, left her standing
all alone.

Nice. That was the thing
in our family, that I should
be nice—no matter what else,
the neighbors should know
how nice I was. Be nice,
what a nice girl, how cute.
Tommy, you say?
So when I stood up
in front of all those people
who wanted me to do something
or be someone, I wanted them
to like me and think I was nice
even when I was telling them that
who I was went against everything
they ever believed in or even
when I was telling them to fight,
to believe in themselves
and fight for what they needed,
still I thought they should think
I was nice. Once I told a friend
I thought people should like me
more, since I was basically
nice. Nice? she asked. Nice?
Don't sell yourself short.
You're not nice.

Peace seemed worth having, personal
peace, the place she could go deep
inside herself and not have to listen
to the voices. Sometimes weeding
the garden, writing in a journal, hearing
different music and the call of each bird,
then she felt at peace. But more often
she would hear the voice and remember
her script and so she would answer
and go and be or do whatever
was required.

And when she had to shut
them out she drank and when she had to go
out to meet them she drank and when
she drank she thought it was they who
would not let her in.
                    So that the rooms
grew darker and the air she breathed seemed
to have all been breathed before.

I shook all day of the night
I went to talk about how maybe
I was ready to think about
not drinking. I'd been alone
for two weeks, told myself I didn't
have a problem. Others made it up.
And if no one was there to see
I'd find my natural level. I did.
And couldn't breathe at all when
I woke up. I was scared.
Scared. I didn't know why
but I was shaking inside and it
worked its way out to my hands
and my voice when I spoke. All day
I said, hey, it's nothing to be
afraid of, and I was afraid.
I'd thought that death was the end
of changing, but this change
felt like death.

Later she would put the lies in here too
but she hadn't gotten that far then—
couldn't see how she'd found the peace
by lying. She used the lies to shut
them all out, to create a false and private
place, and finally the lies
came between her and the woman sleeping
close, and when she'd reach to touch
her arm, she wasn't sure
who she would find there.

We each come differently to that place
where there is nothing left. We reach out
to touch firm ground and find
we've already gone down further even
than that and there is no room to turn,
to shift, no room to move at all
or breathe. The earth sat on her chest
like yesterday's promises.

> I felt like an animal
> gnawing my own leg
> to get out of the trap
> and the blood tasted
> like metal.

She breathed quietly the mute untested
air of the world in which she woke,
longed for the welcoming songs
without knowing what she longed for,
because she had feared this change
like death and she came—a different
kind of creature—back into this
world where yesterday today and tomorrow
were supposed to be the same, a world
in which the old ways were the good ways,
and yet for her the old ways led
only to that place where there was nothing
left and when she came to that place
she knew it now for what it was
and turning she began the journey out.

The Earthquake

I sat up waking
and felt newness
in the still darkened
air   then the earth
trembled   not tentative
but a deepdown rumble
was shaking every surface
and I felt the rocks
shifting and my house
rattling as the earth's
bones readjusted.

When it was quiet
I thought   now they will see
the surface all the same
but underneath I know
every rock and fissure
each line of stress and weakness
has been rearranged and lives
in new relationship   each to each.

Chassé par Terre

One foot after
the other down
into the earth
she followed this
woman who had
journeyed here each
year   naked they
walked to the source
through damp tunnels
hearing the drip
of water the
echo of her
breath   she walked
to the wellspring
waded into
pools   rested thighs
on warm rock   spread
her hair   floating
on the water.

Striated rivers of rock
flowed in colors through the walls
her fingers followed the bump
and ridge of rock memory
and her eyes followed the women
who walked up and down narrow
rock tunnels   dipped into steaming
pools   her eyes followed the planes
and hollows of flesh from which
children had swum and she thought
how rocks held the memory
in fossil of what life there
had been before and how women's
bodies held the memory
of birth and labor in each
muscle and in sagging breasts
and she rested her hand
on her friend's arm   feeling:
the cords of wood split
the child carried and fed
the caress

and she thought how
each loss and pain
must rest in her
like the fossil
not an emblem
of what had been
but the present
moment transformed
always by what
has been   pushing
back to become
part of what is.

The Flowers

She gave them to me with a smile
and said to write a poem about
anemones   I said poems weren't
made that way   smiled   carried them
out to my car where the furious
color of tight anemone buds
mocked the early winter dark.

And so I became a woman
with anemones furled tight
on stems borne down by the weight
of all that color   carmine   lilac
amethyst heads stretched above emerald
leaves curled in a loose fist beneath
the blooms. When one stem bent

and the flower lay limp on the table
I plucked it from the vase
and stuffed it without thought
into the trash where an hour later
I retrieved the stem and flattened
petals. Chastened at last by her
admonition   I imagined these quartz-

clear colors against the clean
falling wet snow   imagined the ceremony
imagined laying the eight spent blooms
together under the boughbent lilac
tree to keep company with the winter
chickadee   and did.   Now I
have been a woman with anemones

who saw (like the painter who gave
the gift) the necessity of ceremony
in colors so deep and clear
the empty ache of a still room
focused and pulled to center
around their presence
who remembers the shadow of colors

on the snow as the lilac branches
loosened and the chickadee eyed
this brilliant intrusion   who lives
in a room where there has been more
than today   who knows no loss
is pure loss

for I remember carmine
on the snow and face
the center of a room
empty with potential.

Lebenstanz

Is *there a* lebenstanz? No *no.*
That is the work we do every day.

In a blizzard she climbed
the hill   wind sucking
at her breath and the snow
icing against her eyes
as she bent her head to walk
forward on instinct
when she could not see
the ground.

In the wind and in the trees
she could hear children's voices
playing and she knew them
as the hill knew the children
who had played here summers
for a hundred years and she heard
their voices laughing in the sharp
teeth of the wind.

The wind left no footprints
but twisted the snow
in wraiths of movement
each dancing on the nothing
below   and the trees bent—
their voices sharp with pain
—and louder than it all
she heard her own heart beating.

To act or not to act
she climbed to find the answer
and in the climbing knew
the answer was to act as though
there were no choice   for if
she believed in the circle—
that as the fossil sinks then
it will rise again to the surface

so all energy comes around
—she must act as though
each day knew the circle   knew
the answer in the wind's sharp voice.
Some days she could only half believe
some days she would know it held no truth
but on the best days she worked as though
the question mattered not at all.

Coming Back

We Pull Off The Road Just Past Amarillo

We pull off the road just past Amarillo
at anywhere Texas a red dirt road
divides the horizon   hiccups over
a railroad crossing and goes on forever.

My jogging shoes follow the lacechain track
of birds—ground nesters I guess—
scanning the fields there is no tree
anywhere and I can see tomorrow.

I run away from the car toward the tracks.
New York plates. Two women running.
I imagine a cop standing by the car
when we return—a fantasy for sure—
out here I couldn't run far enough
to lose sight of the car.

You girls scared? No. I am not running
because I am scared. The sky out here
is so wide I could fall up into it
if I were to lift both feet off the ground
but this does not scare me. And authority
does not scare me today. Though I have never
been anywhere I could tell the good guys
from the bad.

At night we bed down close to the earth
and she pulls me back from the sky
and sometimes it is this that scares me
being this close to the earth.

Politically Incorrect

On the night your lover
takes another lover   theory
takes a back seat and something
right down deep in the gut
centered between your liver
and your self-esteem shoots
bile out into your whole system
and makes you even more
unloveable than you already
have reason to feel.

As nausea clamps down and settles
in for a long stay you have
to realize she didn't get there
(you don't want to think where
just now) by herself and reluctantly
you have to admit you agreed
that too tight a relationship
could stifle individual growth
that after these many years
(how many doesn't seem to matter)
you may be relying a little
more on ritual than spontaneity
but tonight ritual—you remember—
holds many virtues.

It is probably easier if your lover
takes another lover while you
are out of town since nothing
not the anguished silence you
hold on your end of the expensive
long distance phone call
not the silence of a whole
city echoing around you on this
Saturday night when everyone else
is in love or at least in lust
nothing is quite like lying
alone in your double-bed wondering
whether she will choose to come
home or stay away.

And on the morning after your lover
has taken another lover you can hold
meaningful conversations about
what this means to your relationship
and she can tell you she is taking
one day at a time and while you
are theoretically pleased she
is making sure her needs are met
you still taste the vomit
in your throat from the night before
and wonder if all of your friends
find you as unattractive
as your lover.

You have read all the theory
about non-monogamy and how tight
dyads are politically stifling
a real drag in an anarcha-feminist
community but you still can't quite
make yourself go to the meeting
you had planned on for weeks
even if the program material falls
through a crack and your lover
tells you her sex life has nothing
to do with this meeting
but still you can't make yourself
sit down in the same room with them
as though nothing had happened
as though none of the boundaries
had shifted, no fissures had opened
and you had not fallen
through the crack.

What you want to know on this
morning is where are the stories
that tell how it feels to live
right now in your gut not your
head and how long it will be
until you can ask her how are you
and want to know the answer
and whether women die
from this or what percentage
of relationships bite the dust after
this transition from theoretical
to actual non-monogamy.

And when you ask if she means
to still be your lover she says
she expects to have an ongoing
relationship with you and you
will have to decide whether
it matters that she has more
or better orgasms with her new
lover or if you can stop imagining
she is comparing your technique
like a clinician scoring
a novice somewhere deep down
inside that insecurity about
our sexuality so many of us
carry around and when you mumble
something about trust and being
able to let the feeling through
she tells you that you
will have to decide about that.

Still you admit she didn't
get there by herself and you want
to be able to love her and you want
to feel her love coming back at you
but the wires seem tangled
there's another voice on the line
singing   haha   haha   got you
you fool.

It Is In The End A Private Grief

It is in the end a private grief
quiet as a sunset   unheralded
and like nothing you ever expected.

(A woman kneels sweating in the garden
to weed a long row and each time she pulls
the top off a weed and misses the root
she knows she will have to do the job
over again in a day or two).

When a life together hemorrhages
and nothing will stanch the wound
you can hold your hands
to catch the flow   but most
will spill out on the ground.
Days later you will look at the stain
on your hands in wonder.

Adrenaline carries you for seven days
throat dry with fear
hand taut to control the tremor
just when you believe
you will never sleep again
the weight of it crushes you down and down.

In a room   a single shaft
of light does not push back the shadows.
You remember when darkness
was a familiar
and wait each night for the weight
to lift as the sun fades.

Coming Back

for Audre Lorde

Out of these winter depths
a voice summons me:
the only pain that is unbearable
is wasted pain   always there is
something to be learned. I flinch
step back from this voice
that would take me
to the hard places.

I tell you now
I am afraid.

Ice was on the road   ice
was building in the stream
and drooping from the boughs
of every tree as the structure
of my familiar world
seemed to stretch
and then collapse.

Ice bends the white birch into a bow
under its weight   the tree
broken   glittering   in the deceptive
beauty of winter   will not grow
straight up after the thaw.

I became that Minnesota woman
trapped in a nightmare of failure
of risks not visible   when unprotected
and alone at sixty below zero
like her I walked   slowing
toward a destination I could never reach.
The wind shrilled under my short coat
and I slowed   as I walked
each foot a separate effort
the only sound within.

On that icebound road I watched
my stiffening body   how my shoulders
ceased to sway as outside
the earth accelerated   stars kaleidoscoped
seemed to move so fast each path merged
ribbons of light to my slowing eye
past and future slid on the iced wind
as I moved within   as I seemed
to be not here to those outside.

I could have let go
felt the sharpness grow numb
released the pain   walked away
from what I once knew
walked that road swept clean
by wind and snow as though
no one had been here before
as though a voice were not echoing
the only pain that is unbearable
is wasted pain.

if there were silence
if the only voice was the wind's voice
if I pulled all sensation back within
I could begin
the letting go.

But today I choose the journey back
acknowledge the damage   anticipate
the painful thaw   not restitution
a recovery more moderate   more slow.
They found her body cordwood stiff
no pulse or breath discernible
and brought her back each step reversed:

the shard of ice melts from behind our eyes
and we must see again and move again
and know again
what we would not choose to know.

She Had Not Expected This Sudden

She had not expected this sudden
thaw   the wet mouth of spring
on her cheek   her thigh   lusty
and raw   at an hour when she
had been sure of the snow
sure the quiet time would linger
before the torrential spring.

Stay   she warned the plants
and deep-rooted bulbs   stay
she felt danger in the quickening
light and in the sap-starting
warmth   don't move
against the season   stay.

And yet she opened   wet
like summer rain   she opened like
a windblown jonquil   nodding
serenely at the edge of a crusted
snow melting from the rim
of a hill   joyfully   she opened.

Barn Swallows

At the waterfall
were swallows darting
in and around
down to the still surface
of the pool to catch
bugs or play
with a shadow.

When I was a child   said my friend
I lived on a farm and in the spring
the barn swallows would find molted
feathers and play a game on the pond,
flying up, dropping
the feather into
a breeze, then
swooping to pluck it
off the surface of the pond.

Joy   she said   such joy
in their game. And she
was sure it was a game
—a game that taught young
birds to swoop   climb
dive into life.

And I saw then
the awe-filled child who understood
and the adult who remembered

both—
the joy in the bird's self-skill and mastery
the joy of a child, seeing and knowing and praising—

and the gift of the moment returned
when needed   floating
a feather on still water.

Notes

In Greek *metamorphosis* means a marked change in appearance, structure, or function. In English it also carries the connotation of transformation, as by magic or sorcery, in other words an inexplicable change.

Chassé en l'air and *chassé par terre* are ballet dance steps which mean "one foot follows the other in the air" and "one foot follows the other on the earth."

Totentanz and *lebenstanz* mean, literally, death dance and life dance.

Other titles from Firebrand Books include:

The Big Mama Stories by Shay Youngblood/$8.95

A Burst of Light, Essays by Audre Lorde/$7.95

Diamonds Are A Dyke's Best Friend by Yvonne Zipter/$9.95

Dykes To Watch Out For, Cartoons by Alison Bechdel/$6.95

The Fires Of Bride, A Novel by Ellen Galford/$8.95

A Gathering Of Spirit, A Collection by North American Women edited by Beth Brant (*Degonwadonti*)/$9.95

Getting Home Alive by Aurora Levins Morales and Rosario Morales /$8.95

Good Enough To Eat, A Novel by Lesléa Newman/$8.95

Jonestown & Other Madness, Poetry by Pat Parker/$5.95

The Land Of Look Behind, Prose and Poetry by Michelle Cliff /$6.95

A Letter To Harvey Milk, Short Stories by Lesléa Newman/$8.95

Letting In The Night, A Novel by Joan Lindau/$8.95

Living As A Lesbian, Poetry by Cheryl Clarke/$6.95

Making It, A Woman's Guide to Sex in the Age of AIDS by Cindy Patton and Janis Kelly/$3.95

Mohawk Trail by Beth Brant (*Degonwadonti*)/$6.95

Moll Cutpurse, A Novel by Ellen Galford/$7.95

More Dykes To Watch Out For, Cartoons by Alison Bechdel/$7.95

The Monarchs Are Flying, A Novel by Marion Foster/$8.95

My Mama's Dead Squirrel, Lesbian Essays on Southern Culture by Mab Segrest/$8.95

Politics Of The Heart, A Lesbian Parenting Anthology edited by Sandra Pollack and Jeanne Vaughn/$11.95

Presenting . . . Sister NoBlues by Hattie Gossett/$8.95

A Restricted Country by Joan Nestle/$8.95

Sanctuary, A Journey by Judith McDaniel/$7.95

Shoulders, A Novel by Georgia Cotrell/$8.95

The Sun Is Not Merciful, Short Stories by Anna Lee Walters/$7.95

Tender Warriors, A Novel by Rachel Guido deVries/$7.95

This Is About Incest by Margaret Randall/$7.95

The Threshing Floor, Short Stories by Barbara Burford/$7.95

Trash, Stories by Dorothy Allison/$8.95

The Women Who Hate Me, Poetry by Dorothy Allison/$5.95

Words To The Wise, A Writer's Guide to Feminist and Lesbian Periodicals & Publishers by Andrea Fleck Clardy/$3.95

Yours In Struggle, Three Feminist Perspectives on Anti-Semitism and Racism by Elly Bulkin, Minnie Bruce Pratt, and Barbara Smith/$8.95

You can buy Firebrand titles at your bookstore, or order them directly from the publisher (141 The Commons, Ithaca, New York 14850, 607-272-0000).

Please include $1.75 shipping for the first book and $.50 for each additional book.

A free catalog is available on request.